YOGA TO BUILD STRENGTH

Elevate Your Fitness and Well-Being

Steven m. Bowman

1

Table of contents

Introduction

Welcome to the world of "Yoga to Build Strength"! In the pages that follow, you will embark on a journey to harness the transformative power of yoga, specifically tailored to help you cultivate physical strength, mental resilience, and inner balance.

In a world filled with complex fitness routines and high-intensity workouts, we often overlook the profound simplicity and effectiveness of yoga. This book is your entry point into a practice that not only

Table Of Contents

Introduction

What is going on with the human way of behaving?
Conduct alludes to your activities or responses in light of
inward or outer boost circumstances. Brain research
comprehends the idea of the human way of behaving, which is
anything an individual does and clinicians can notice, record,
and measure it. You can comprehend an individual's way of
behaving when you know the reasons that caused the
individual to act how they do or their reaction in case of
something occurring. By endorsing or disliking conduct, you
assess conduct, which happens every day for the vast
majority.

For what reason do people act how they do?
People act how they do given their temperament and sustain,
which is the idea of the psychosocial climate. In making sense
of a human way of behaving, the natural viewpoint
distinguishes hereditary qualities, development, chemicals,
and DNA makeup as assuming a critical part in significantly
shaping the human way of behaving. A phenomenal
illustration of how hereditary qualities assume an urgent part
in molding characters, particularly for those related, is in
twins, who, in any event, when isolated, show comparative

characteristics. You know how hereditary inclinations shape your conduct by seeing how your folks, kin, and different family members act.

The sustained viewpoint makes sense of conduct as being formed by the psychosocial climate, however, individuals have some control over their way of behaving. In support, the psychosocial climate incorporates childhood, friends, and present environmental elements. There are numerous instances of the impacts of support on conduct that can assist you with figuring out individuals' way of behaving, for example, crediting ways of behaving and issues to youth and guardians molding their kids' future. Likewise, peers impact individuals' ways of behaving and may change depending upon their exercises and conditions

Chapter 1

Four essential kinds of characters in the human way of behaving

The four essential kinds of human characters in the human way of behaving are jealous, hopeful, cynical, and trusting. Since the four particular characters exist in every single individual, you display unmistakable characters in various circumstances. Likewise, character types have a few equilibria and an individual might show a character type and its contrary side, contingent upon the circumstance. The following are the four kinds of characters in the human way of behaving:

Jealous
Individuals with a jealous character frequently try to be preferable over every other person, regardless of the accomplishment. When confronted with choices, they pick a choice that makes them comparable to their accomplices or stunningly better than them. You can in any case be steady, in any event, when you have this character.

Hopeful
Individuals with a hopeful character generally have trust that everything might pan out in all circumstances and continue, during convoluted circumstances. They trust others can go with the most ideal choices very much like them and select

the most ideal choices. However, you might be a hopeful person, and a few circumstances might make you critical.

Critical
Critical individuals feel a little unsure about nearly all that and frequently pick the least damaging options when they have choices. As a worrier, you select choices that guarantee you some triumph instead of those that might prompt losing. You may likewise be hopeful in specific circumstances since the character types have an equilibrium of some sort or another.

Trusting
Individuals with this character trust others without requiring significant motivation to trust them. They help out others and wouldn't fret about the result, like winning or losing. With a believing character, you work together with your accomplice without reconsidering; however, there are a few circumstances in which may generally doubt others, for example, when they deceive you several

Chapter 2

Characteristics Of The Four Sorts of the Human Way of Behaving

Exploring Logical, Affable, Expressive, and Driver Characters

Understanding the subtleties of the human way of behaving requires a more critical gander at the particular originals that frequently arise in different social settings. These paradigms act as layouts for how people process data, simply decide, and interface with others. In this part, we dive into the complexities of the four essential conduct types - the Logical Scholar, the Genial Ally, the Expressive Powerhouse, and the Driver Chief.

2.1 The Insightful Mastermind

Attributes:

Conscious and thorough way to deal with errands
An inclination for information-driven direction
Saved disposition and accentuation on exactness
Correspondence Procedures:

Giving exhaustive information and proof to help contentions
Permitting time for insightful examination before anticipating a reaction
Recognizing their meticulousness and accuracy

2.2 The Affable Ally

Attributes:

Accentuation on keeping up with agreeable connections
Regular tendency towards sympathy and participation
Patient and obliging attitude
Correspondence Techniques:

Making a warm and cordial air
Recognizing their commitments to the group and esteeming their feedback
Permitting space for open conversations and communicating sentiments

2.3 The Expressive Powerhouse

Qualities:

Magnetic and convincing in their collaborations

Blossom with social commitment and associations
Excited and hopeful viewpoint
Correspondence Systems:

Taking part in enthusiastic and dynamic discussions
Permitting potential opens doors for them to communicate
innovativeness and thoughts
Perceiving their capacity to rouse and spur others

2.4 **The Driver Chief**

Qualities:

Results-situated and objective-driven
Emphatic and p, positive about the direction
The normal tendency to win influential
Correspondence Procedures:

Zeroing in on goals, results, and activity plans
Giving clear assumptions and cutoff times
Recognizing their drive and assurance in accomplishing
objectives
By unwinding the interesting characteristics and inclinations
of every conduct type, we gain important bits of knowledge
about how people process data and move toward difficulties.
Furnished with this information, we are better prepared to
tailor our correspondence styles to successfully draw in
Logical Scholars, Friendly Allies, Expressive Powerhouses,
and Driver Pioneers in a way that resounds with their
unmistakable characters.

Chapter 3

Perceiving Conduct Types

Interpreting circumstances

While understanding the hypothetical structure of conduct types is critical, the genuine worth lies in its application in certifiable situations.... This part conquers any issues between theory and work, offering significant models and context-oriented examinations that show how lead types manifest in various settings.....

3.1 Contextual investigations: Unwinding Ways of behaving

Situation 1: The Group Task

Investigating how to conduct types impact group elements and direction
Recognizing possible contentions and utilizing qualities for ideal results

Situation 2: Client Collaboration

Exploring client connections by perceiving and adjusting to
their conduct types
Exhibiting how compelling correspondence prompts fruitful
client collaborations

3.2 Distinguishing Prevailing Ways of Behaving

Perception Procedures:

Perceiving verbal signs, non-verbal communication, and
correspondence styles characteristic of conduct types
Understanding how people answer difficulties and express
inclinations

Appraisal Devices and Studies:

Investigating approved instruments for evaluating conduct
types
Utilizing self-evaluation and companion appraisal for
thorough bits of knowledge

3.3 Fitting Systems for Explicit Settings

Initiative and The executives:

Adjusting correspondence styles to lead and propel different
conduct types
Developing a fair group dynamic through essential
designation
Compromise:

Utilizing con bass experiences in intervenes clashes and track down commonly advantageous arrangements
Keeping miscommunication from growing into bigger issues
By drenching ourselves in viable models and methods, we gain a more profound appreciation for the nuanced ways conduct types impact our collaborations. Through sharp discernment, evaluation, and essential variety, we get ready for extra pleasant and helpful associations in both master and individual circles.

Chapter 4

Fitting Correspondence Styles

Adjusting and Redoing Correspondence for Mosthe t extreme Effect

Powerful correspondence is a unique cycle that requires versatility and adaptability. Perceiving the variety of conduct types, we should adjust our way of dealing with interfaces seriously with people across the range...... this section, we explore methods for fitting correspondence styles to resonate with Logical Brains, Charming Partners, Expressive Forces to be reckoned with, and Driver Trailblazers...

4.1 Adaptability in Correspondence

Versatile Language and Tone:

Balancing language intricacy and convention a in given crowd's conduct type

Tweaking tone to line up with the singular's inclinations for certainty or warmth

Adaptability in Medium:

Utilizing different correspondence channels (e.g., composed, verbal, visual) to take care of assorted inclinations

Perceiving when eye-to-eye connections are liked over advanced correspondence

4.2 Adjusting to Various Sorts

Logical Masterminds:

Giving itemized, efficient data with accentuation on precision and dependability

Permitting time for reflection and questions, regarding their requirement for accuracy

Pleasant Allies:

Laying out trust and compatibility through open, amicable, and sympathetic correspondence

Esteeming their feedback and effectively standing by listening to their interests, guaranteeing they feel appreciated and comprehended

Expressive Forces to be reckoned with:

Taking part in powerful, lively discussions that consider imagination and thought age

Recognizing their energy and giving open doors to them to share their vision

Driver Pioneers:

Arriving at the point rapidly, zeroing in on results, and framing clear activity steps

Showing certainty and confidence while regarding their time requirements

4.3 Calibrating Correspondence for Explicit Settings

Gatherings and Introductions:

Fitting substance and conveyance to suit the inclinations of different conduct types in participation

Guaranteeing that data is introduced such that requests to scientific, friendly, expressive, and driver characters

Dealings and Deals:

Adjusting exchange procedures to line up with the correspondence style of the partner

Building trust and compatibility by perceiving and tending to the requirements and needs of every conduct type

Administration and The executives:

Utilizing conduct-based correspondence to read and lead assorted groups

Perceiving when to apply decisiveness or compassion in given conduct types included

By prevailing at fitting correspondence styles, we open the potential for extra huge affiliations, dealt with joint effort, and more important results. This adaptable method licenses us to rise above deterrent relationships with people of all lead types.

Chapter 5

Conquering Correspondence Difficulties

Exploring Struggle, Opposition, and Boundaries to Compelling Correspondence

Compelling correspondence isn't without its difficulties... Disarrays, clashes, and locks can emerge, particularly while administering organized direct sorts. In this piece, we address commonly normal obstacles and give structures to conquering them, guaranteeing smooth and obliging joint endeavors.

5.1 Managing Struggle

Perceiving the Indications of Contention:

Distinguishing conduct prompts demonstrating possible struggles
Understanding how different conduct types express disappointment or conflict
Useful Compromise:

Carrying out undivided attention and compassion to see all points of view

Cooperatively tracking down eye-to-eye that considers the requirements of all gatherings included
Intervening and Working with:

Using conduct-based bits of knowledge to intercede clashes between people with various correspondence styles
Establishing a climate helpful for open and deferential discourse

5.2 carsharing car care Opposition

Figuring out Wellsprings of Opposition:

Investigating how conduct types might answer distinctively to change or novel thoughts
Distinguishing triggers for obstruction and tending to them proactively
Acquiring Purchase In and Participation:

Fitting correspondence to address the worries and needs of people with changing conduct types
Features advantages and adjusting objectives to cultivate collaboration

5.3 Tending to Correspondence Hindrances

Language and Phrasing:

Keeping away from language or complex language that might estrange specific conduct types

Guaranteeing clearness and shared figuring out through worked on correspondence

Non-Verbal Correspondence:

Focusing on non-verbal communication, signals, and looks to measure openness
Adjusting non-verbal signals to the favored correspondence style of the person

5.4 Developing a Culture of Compelling Correspondence

Influential positions:

Displaying viable correspondence ways of behaving for the group
Laying out clear correspondence assumptions and giving assets to expertise advancement
Criticism and Ceaseless Improvement:

Requesting input from colleagues to evaluate correspondence adequacy
Carrying out methodologies for progressing improvement and expert turn of events
By proactively tending to and exploring difficulties in correspondence, we establish a climate where different conduct types can team up amicably, at last prompting more effective results in both business and individual associations.

Chapter 6

Building Powerful Groups

Utilizing Different Conduct Types for Ideal Execution

A durable and high-performing group is the foundation of any effective undertaking. Understanding the different direct sorts inside a social occasion gives a supportive asset for furnishing individual qualities and spreading out synergistic workblocks In this portion, we explore strategies for social occasions and driving gatherings that bloom with the clever responsibilities of Logical Researchers, Friendly Partners, Expressive Forces to be reckoned with, and Driver Trailblazers...

6.1 Corresponding Conduct Types

Perceiving Cooperative energies:

Distinguishing how the qualities of one conduct type supplement the shortcomings of another
Utilizing these collaborations to upgrade group execution and critical thinking capacities
Adjusting Ranges of abilities:

Guaranteeing that every conduct type contributes its specific abilities to the group's general goals and capacities

6.2 Encouraging Coordinated

Establishing a Comprehensive Climate:

Empowering open and common regard among colleagues
with fluctuating conduct types
Esteeming and praising the assorted points of view and
approaches every part offers of real value

Characterizing jobs in light of people's assets and inclinations
Putting forth clear execution assumptions and objectives to
direct the group toward progress.

6.3 Authority and Direction

Adjusting Authority Styles:

Fitting authority ways to deal with suit the necessities and
correspondence styles of colleagues
Offering the fundamental help and direction for every conduct
type to succeed in their jobs
Enabling Colleagues:

Confiding in people to take responsibility for obligations and
pursue choices inside their subject matters
Offering open doors for expertise advancement and
development in light of conduct types qualities.

6.4 Exploring Difficulties in Inside

Compromise and Intercession:

Using conduct-sexperiences to address clashes and cultivate useful goals
Going about as a middle person to guarantee all voices are heard and concerns are tended to.

Keeping up with Inspiration and Confidence:

Perceiving the inspirational drivers of every conduct type and giving custom-made motivating forces and input
Establishing a positive workplace that upholds the prosperity and occupation fulfillment of all colleagues
By deliberately utilizing the qualities and correspondence styles of different conduct types, we encourage a dynamic and successful group that meets its objectives as well as flourishes in its cooperative undertakings.

Chapter 7

Correspondence Strategies for Explicit Situations

Applying Conduct-Based Correspondence in Key Business Circumstances

In different expert situations, the capacity to convey actually can have a significant effect on progress and botched open doors. This part jumps into custom-fitted correspondence philosophies for unequivocal settings, ensuring that Shrewd Brains, Pleasant Partners, Expressive Forces to be reckoned with, and Driver Trailblazers are secured and responsive.

7.1 Gatherings and Introductions

Readiness and Content Design:

Adjusting the substance and design of introductions to take care of various conduct types

Guaranteeing that data is introduced in a reasonable, coordinated way for Scientific Masterminds, and in a connecting way for Expressive Powerhouses.

Commitment and Interest:

Empowering dynamic support from all conduct types through designated assistance methods
Giving chances to open conversations while guaranteeing that all voices are heard and esteemed

7.2 Exchanges and Deals

Understanding Client Conduct Types:

Breaking down client conduct to tailor exchange and deal methodologies
Tending to worries and featuring benefits in a manner that reverberates with every conduct type.

Building Trust and Affinity:

Laying out areas of strength for Arusttrustugh successful correspondence and comprehension of client inclinations
Exhibiting a veritable interest in addressing the requirements and assumptions of clients

7.3 Adminithe Board and The Board

Course and Objective Setting:

Giving clear headings and assumptions that line up with the objectives and correspondence styles of colleagues
Guaranteeing that targets are conveyed in a way that reverberates with every conduct type

Criticism and Acknowledgment:

Fitting input and acknowledgment techniques to suit the inclinations of people with various conduct types
Recognizing and commending accomplishments in a manner that propels and motivates colleagues

7.4 Emergency Correspondence and Troublesome Discussions

Keeping calm and Lucidity:

Applying conduct-based bits of knowledge to stay created and articulate during high-stress circumstances
Conveying troublesome messages with compassion and impressive skill
Settling on some shared interests:

Utilizing conduct-based correspondence to recognize shared objectives and interests, even in testing conditions
Looking for commonly advantageous arrangements through open discourse and cooperation
By fitting correspondence methods to explicit business situations, we upgrade our capacity to interface with people of all conduct types, eventually prompting more fruitful results and more grounded proficient connections.

Chapter 8

Self-awareness and Improvement

Saddling Conduct-Based Correspondence for Personal Growth

Successful correspondence isn't just about grasping others; it's likewise about perceiving and fostering our correspondence style. In this part, we analyze how seeing our lead type and further fostering our correspondence limits can incite self-improvement and seriously convincing facilitated endeavors.

8.1 Perceiving Your Conduct Type

Self-Appraisal and Reflection:

Taking part in thoughtfulness to distinguish our conduct propensities and correspondence inclinations
Using evaluation devices and criticism from peers for an exhaustive comprehension
Embracing Qualities and Tending to Shortcomings:

Commending our novel assets and involving them for our potential benefit in expert and individual settings

Recognizing regions for development and looking for open doors for development

8.2 Further developing Relational abilities

Undivided attention and Sympathy:

Developing undivided attention abilities to all the more likely figure out the viewpoints and necessities of others
Creating compassion as a way to interface on a more profound level and fabricate trust

Adjusting Correspondence Styles:

Rehearsing adaptability in correspondence to reverberate with various conduct types
Figuring out how to change tone, and language, and move toward given the inclinations of our crowd.

8.3 Improving Compromise Capacities

Staying cool and Goal:

Building the ability to understand people on a deeper level to explore clashes with self-control and fairness
Zeroing in on finding commonly helpful arrangements as opposed to appointing fault

Arranging Mutual Benefit Results:

Using relational abilities to work with useful discussions and agree

Offsetting emphaticness with a cooperative methodology for ideal outcomes.

8.4 Laying out and Accomplishing Individual Objectives

Adjusting Objectives to Conduct Type Qualities:

Utilizing conduct-based experiences to put forth objectives that line up with our normal tendencies and qualities

Expanding our true capacity for progress by gaining what comes most normally

Following Advancement and Observing Achievements:

Carrying out procedures for estimating and celebrating individual accomplishments

Perceiving the worth of little triumphs in the excursion toward bigger goals

By zeroing in on our conduct type and refining our relational abilities, we not only improve our capacity to associate with others but also enable ourselves to develop expertly.

Chapter 9

Social Responsiveness in Correspondence

Exploring Different Social Settings for Successful Cooperation

In the present interconnected worldwide scene, understanding and regarding social contrasts is fundamental for fruitful correspondence. This part dives into the meaning of social mindfulness and gives procedures for changing correspondence styles to suit grouped social circumstances…

9.1 Adjusting to Assorted Workplaces

Social Mindfulness and Awareness:

Fostering an increased consciousness of social subtleties, values, and customs is basic to powerful culturally diverse correspondence. This includes investigating, going to social studios, and partaking in open conversations with individuals from different establishments. It's fundamental to push toward each coordinated effort with a genuine interest and excitement to learn.

Perceiving possible areas of social misconception or confusion is similarly urgent. Certain movements, tones, or even kinds of addresses could hold different ramifications in various social orders. A careful methodology guarantees that unexpected tactless acts are stayed away from.

Regarding Customs and Practices:

Exhibiting regard for neighborhood customs, ceremonies, and behaviors says a lot about one's social responsiveness. This might include adjusting clothing, good tidings, or gift-giving practices to line up with the social standards of the climate. By showing an interest in and regard for the social texture, people can construct affinity and trust in the local area.

In like manner, understanding the significance of unequivocal practices can affect more essential affiliations... For example, partaking in common exercises or services can open doors for more profound associations and a more extravagant comprehension of the social setting.

9.2 Keeping Away from Misconceptions

Explaining Assumptions and Goals:

Guaranteeing that messages are passed on with clearness and accuracy is especially basic in multifaceted cooperations. It's fundamental to stay away from presumptions and give more than adequate settings to guarantee common comprehension. This could incorporate presenting genuine requests, searching for clarification, and summarizing focal issues to assert understanding.

Looking for data and demand is an important asset for confirming a common point of view. Empowering people to share their understanding of the message guarantees

arrangement as well as exhibits a pledge to successful correspondence.

Receptiveness to Input and Transformation:

A genuinely socially delicate communicator is available to get criticism and will adjust their correspondence style in light of the experiences acquired. This might include effectively looking for criticism from people inside the social setting and integrating it into future associations. It's a continuous course of learning and adjusting to guarantee that correspondence stays powerful and conscious.

9.3 Utilizing Variety for Development and Development

Saddling Alternate points of view:

Perceiving the improving capability of different social foundations in critical thinking and development is a foundation of viable culturally diverse joint efforts. By esteeming various perspectives and approaches, groups can show up at additional thorough and creative arrangements. This variety of thought drives innovativeness and encourages a climate of ceaseless learning.

Encouraging a comprehensive climate where all voices are esteemed and heard is fundamental. This might include making stages for open exchange, celebrating social celebrations, and giving open doors to workers to share their interesting social encounters. ..In doing so, associations can take advantage of an abundance of imagination and skill…

Advancing a Culture of Incorporation:

Pushing for methodologies and practices that back and embrace assortment is a basic stage toward laying out a complete work environment. This might include carrying out racial awareness schooling programs, laying out mentorship drives, and guaranteeing equivalent admittance to open doors for all workers. By propelling inclusivity, affiliations foster a culture where individuals feel regarded and connected to contribute their wonderful perspectives. Giving assets and amazing chances for culturally diverse learning and improvement is another key viewpoint. This could incorporate language courses, social trade projects, and discussions for sharing encounters. Such drives work with self-improvement as well as fortify the by and large social skill of the association.

9.4 Moral Contemplations in Diverse Correspondence

Regarding Social Limits and Values:

Guaranteeing that correspondence lines up with the moral norms and upsides of the separate culture is of foremost significance. This includes staying away from ways of behaving or language that may unintentionally outrage or discourtesy social responsive qualities. It's urgent to lead a thorough investigation and search for bearing while at the same time investigating conceivably sensitive focuses or conditions. Sticking to social standards likewise stretches out to regions like clothing regulation, dependability, and

gift-giving decorum. Understanding and regarding these subtleties exhibits an elevated degree of social mindfulness and gains appreciation and trust from people inside the social setting.

Developing Trust and Common Regard:

Building trust by exhibiting realness, uprightness, and a certified interest in understanding different viewpoints is central to compelling multifaceted correspondence. This includes undivided attention, showing sympathy, and getting some margin to assemble significant connections. It's fundamental to center around relationship-working over trades, as trust approaches the bedrock of powerful different joint efforts.

Esteeming the commitments and encounters of people from various social foundations is a fundamental part of common regard. Perceiving and commending variety encourages a climate where all colleagues feel seen, heard, and esteemed for their extraordinary viewpoints and commitments.

By zeroing in on friendly responsiveness and changing correspondence styles to suit grouped group environments, we develop an environment of inclusivity, shared respect, and reasonable correspondence, in the long run provoking more grounded overall affiliations and helpful endeavors.

Chapter 10

Contextual analyses::Applying Behavior-Based Correspondence.

Genuine Instances of Examples of Overcoming Adversity

Gaining from pragmatic models is a strong method for understanding how conduct-based correspondence techniques can be applied in different situations. This part presents a choice of contextual analyses that grandstand effective executions of conduct-based correspondence in different expert settings.

10.1 Contextual Analysis 1:
Worldwide Group Cooperation

Situation:
A worldwide organization with groups scattered across various landmasses confronted moves in cooperation due to social and correspondence boundaries.

Approach:
The association executed diverse preparation for colleagues, zeroing in on conduct-based correspondence procedures. This remembered studios for social mindfulness, undivided attention, and adjusting correspondence styles.

Result:

By perceiving and regarding the conduct of colleagues from various social foundations, the groups had the option to impart all the more. This incited better participation, extended proficiency, and a more pleasing work environment.

10.2 Contextual analysis

2: Client Relationship The board Situation:

A counseling firm attempted to lay areas of strength for our connections, as their correspondence style didn't necessarily in all cases line up with the inclinations of their different client base.

Approach:

The firm conducted appraisals for both their colleagues and clients. This gave significant bits of knowledge into the conduct of each party included. They then fitted their correspondence systems to match the inclinations of individual clients.

Result:

The guiding firm saw an enormous improvement in client satisfaction and upkeep. By adjusting their correspondence styles to suit the conduct sorts of every client, they had the option to construct more grounded, more productive connections.

10.3 Contextual investigation

3: Initiative Viability

Situation:

A medium-sized organization confronted difficulties with representative commitment and confidence because of a distinction between initiative and staff.

Approach:
The organization gave authority to prepare the remembered modules for conduct-based correspondence. Pioneers figured out how to perceive and adjust to the conduct of their colleagues, encouraging better comprehension and trust.

Result:
Worker fulfillment scores expanded, and turnover rates diminished. The better correspondence among pioneers and staff prompted a more sure workplace, more significant levels of inspiration, and expanded efficiency.

10.4 Contextual investigation
4: Arranging Global Organizations

Situation:
A startup tried to grow its worldwide reach through organizations with global associations, yet experienced moves in discussions because of social contrasts.

Approach:
The startup's group went through serious social responsiveness preparation, zeroing in on conduct-based correspondence. They additionally enrolled the assistance of neighborhood social counsels to give bits of knowledge into the conduct sorts of expected accomplices.

Result:
The startup successfully settled relationships with relationships in arranged areas. By getting it and adjusting to the conduct sorts of their worldwide partners, they had the option to haggle commonly helpful arrangements and grow their worldwide presence.

By investigating these significant evaluations, people gain principal snippets of data on how noxious correspondence designs can be applied to attested conditions. These examples of overcoming adversity act as motivation for executing comparable methodologies in their proficient collaborations.

Chapter 11

Supporting Powerful Correspondence Practices

Methodologies for Long Haul Achievement

Keeping up with compelling correspondence rehearses requires progressing exertion and a promise to consistent improvement. In this part, we explore strategies for supporting behavior-based correspondence for a long time, ensuring that it remains an underpinning of productive joint efforts in both master and individual circles.

11.1 Persistent Learning and Improvement

Remaining Refreshed on Correspondence Patterns:

Staying informed about arising patterns and best practices in correspondence is fundamental. This might include going to studios, online courses, and meetings, as well as staying aware of significant distributions and industry websites.

Participating in Proficient Advancement Open doors:
Effectively searching out open doors for ability building and expert development, for example, high-level correspondence courses, initiative preparation, and studios zeroed in on relational adequacy.

11.2 Criticism and Reflection

Looking for Customary Input:
Effectively requesting criticism from partners, managers, and colleagues to acquire experiences in correspondence viability. This can be achieved through outlines, one-on-one discussions, or coordinated input gatherings.

Pondering Correspondence Collaborations:
Participating in ordinary self-reflection to evaluate correspondence collaborations and distinguish regions for development. This might include journaling, self-appraisal activities, or looking for input from confided-in tutors or friends.

11.3 Developing a Culture of Powerful Correspondence

Showing others how it's done:

Displaying powerful correspondence ways of behaving for colleagues and partners, exhibiting the worth put on clear, aware, and comprehensive correspondence.

Advancing Open Discourse:
Establishing a climate where transparent correspondence is supported, and where people feel enabled to voice their considerations and concerns.

11.4 Empowering Diverse Encounters

Supporting Diverse Preparation and Trades:
Giving chances to colleagues to take part in multifaceted encounters, for example, global tasks, social submersion projects, or support in different working gatherings.

Working with Variety and Incorporation Drives:
Effectively advancing variety and incorporation inside the association, and perceiving the worth that assorted points of view bring to correspondence elements.

11.5 Utilizing Innovation for Compelling Correspondence

Remaining Informed About Specialized Instruments:
Staying informed concerning the most recent correspondence innovations and stages, and utilizing them to improve correspondence effectiveness and reach.

Preparing on Innovative Instruments:

Giving preparation and assets to colleagues to use specialized apparatuses, is utilized to their maximum capacity to guarantee them.

By executing these systems, people, and associations can lay out a maintainable starting point for conduct-based correspondence.

Chapter 12

Assessing Correspondence Feasibility

Gadgets and Estimations for Studying Correspondence Impact

Evaluating the practicality of correspondence systems is essential for rolling out informed improvements and ensuring tireless improvement.

12.1 Criticism Components

Studies and Criticism Structures:

Overseeing studies to assemble criticism from colleagues, clients, and partners regarding their view of correspondence adequacy. This can consolidate requests regarding clarity, responsiveness, and satisfaction.

Criticism:
Executing a thorough criticism process where people get input from peers, managers, direct reports, and different partners. This multi-perspective methodology gives a reasonable assessment of social abilities.

12.2 Key Execution Markers (KPIs)

Reaction and Commitment Rates:
Checking reaction rates to messages, messages, or introductions to measure how well the correspondence is resounding with the crowd. High reaction rates might demonstrate successful correspondence.

Meeting Participation and Investment:
Following participation and level of support in gatherings and introductions, as dynamic contribution frequently implies commitment and understanding.

12.3 Correspondence Reviews

Content Investigation:
Directing an intensive examination of composed and verbal correspondence materials to evaluate clearness, intelligibility, and arrangement with conduct-based correspondence standards.

Directing Counterfeit Situations:
Reproducing correspondence situations and assessing members' reactions in light of conduct-type experiences.

12.4 Observational Evaluations

Non-verbal Communication and Non-Verbal Signs:
Noticing and investigating non-verbal communication, looks, and other non-verbal signals during correspondence connections to evaluate levels of commitment and understanding.

Undivided attention and Compassion:
Evaluating the capacity to effectively tune in, show compassion, and adjust correspondence styles in light of noticed conduct types.

12.5 Result-Based Assessment

Influence on Business Goals:
Assessing how conduct-based correspondence procedures have added to accomplishing explicit business objectives, like expanded deals, further developed client fulfillment or improved group execution.

Decrease in Struggle and False impressions:
Following are examples of contention or misconception when executing conduct-based correspondence systems to quantify their viability in lessening such events.

By utilizing these gadgets and estimations, individuals and affiliations have significant indirect-correspondence tries. This information-driven approach empowers informed direction and considers designated changes by additional improved correspondence adequacy.

Chapter 13

Adjusting to Impelling Correspondence Models

Remaining Significant in a Changing Correspondence Scene

As innovation and cultural standards keep on developing, so too do the strategies and stages through which we convey. This portion explores methods for staying agile and changing behavior-based correspondence to fulfill the necessities of a continuously changing correspondence scene.

13.1 Embracing Innovative Headways

Staying informed concerning Specialized Apparatuses:
Staying informed about arising correspondence advances, for example, informing applications, coordinated effort stages, and video conferencing devices. Investigating how these instruments can be utilized to upgrade conduct-based correspondence.

Preparing for New Innovations:
Giving preparation and assets to colleagues to successfully use the most recent specialized devices. This guarantees that the association stays on the front line of correspondence rehearses.

13.2 Bridling Virtual Entertainment and Advanced Stages

Grasping Virtual Entertainment Elements:
Perceiving the impact of virtual entertainment on correspondence patterns and understanding how different conduct types draw in with different stages. This data helps the headway concerning committed correspondence systems.

Using Web-based Entertainment for Commitment:
Utilizing stages like LinkedIn, Twitter, and others to share important substance, draw in adherents, and assemble significant expert connections. This expands the range of conduct-based correspondence endeavors.

13.3 Integrating Visual and Interactive Media Components

Visual Narrating:
Perceiving the force of visual correspondence and integrating components like infographics, recordings, and pictures to upgrade the effect of messages, particularly for conduct types that answer well to visual boosts.

Intelligent Introductions and Online Courses:
Planning connecting with intelligent introductions or online classes that take care of various conduct types. This could consolidate overviews, breakout gatherings, and significant entryways for swarm cooperation.

13.4 Adjusting to Remote Work and Virtual Conditions

Streamlining Virtual Correspondence:
Figuring out the remarkable difficulties of virtual correspondence and carrying out methodologies to keep up with commitment and association with colleagues, clients, and partners.

Adjusting Coordinated and Nonconcurrent Correspondence:
Perceiving when coordinated correspondence (e.g., video calls) is fundamental, and when offbeat correspondence (e.g., messages, informing) is more suitable given conduct type inclinations.

13.5 Exploring Crossover Work Models

Adaptability and Customization:

Recognizing the different requirements and inclinations of colleagues in cross-breed workplaces. Considering adaptability in specialized techniques and obliging individual conduct types.

Making Comprehensive Virtual Spaces:
Guaranteeing that virtual gatherings and joint efforts are comprehensive and open to all colleagues, no matter what their area or correspondence style.

By embracing these frameworks, individuals, and affiliations can proactively change in the coming Correspondence scene. This deftness empowers them to stay pertinent, actually draw in different conduct types, and eventually proceed with progress in their expert collaborations.

Chapter 14

Developing a Culture of Persistent Improvement

Encouraging a Development Outlook in Correspondence

A culture of persistent improvement in correspondence is fundamental for long-haul achievement. This section examines procedures for fanning out an environment where individuals are encouraged to foster their social cut-off points and conform to making conditions.

14.1 Empowering Learning and Improvement

Giving Learning Amazing Open Doors:

Offering admittance to studios, workshops, and online courses zeroed in on relational abilities. This urges individuals to place assets into their turn of events and advancement.

Supporting Ability building Drives:
Distributing assets for workers to go to pertinent preparation projects or seek after confirmations that upgrade their correspondence capacities.

14.2 Perceiving and Observing Accomplishments

Recognizing Achievements:
Commending individual and group accomplishments in correspondence. Seeing advancement invigorates pride and develops the value of strong correspondence.

Featuring Examples of overcoming adversity:
Sharing examples of overcoming adversity of people or groups who have succeeded in their correspondence endeavors. This fills in as motivation and gives instances of best practices.

14.3 Giving Helpful Input

Convenient and Explicit Input:
Offering helpful criticism on relational abilities promptly. Giving express models and huge thoughts for improvement. Cultivating a Culture that welcomes inputs:
Establishing a climate where input isn't just acknowledged but is effectively searched out. Empowering open discussions about correspondence qualities and regions for development.

14.4 Advancing Companion Learning and Mentorship

Distributed Information Sharing:
Working with valuable open doors for representatives to impart their correspondence bits of knowledge and encounters to each other. This empowers a supportive learning climate.

Formal Mentorship Projects:
Laying out mentorship programs where experienced communicators can give direction and backing to those hoping to improve their relational abilities.

14.5 Embracing Trial and Error and Development

Empowering Innovative Correspondence Approaches:
Considering trial and error with new specialized strategies and advances. This urges people to start something new and inspect inventive ways to deal with passing on messages.

Gaining from Disappointments:
Making a place of refuge for people to face challenges in their correspondence endeavors. At the point when errors happen, involving them as learning potential opens doors as opposed to wellsprings of analysis.

Via these frameworks, individuals, and affiliations foster a culture of steady improvement in correspondence. This development mentality benefits individual expertise advancement as well as adds to the general achievement and viability of correspondence inside the association.

Chapter 15

Undertaking in Erratic Business areas

15.1 Composed Undertaking:
Driving Advancement in Strong Regions
Bit by bit directions to Encourage an Ambitious Attitude:
Creative and versatile business pioneers succeed. ...They should foster a leading mindset inside the business, enabling progress, continuing reasonable procedures, and shaking the boat..... Bunches with this disposition are more ready to successfully look for possible results and lift advancement due to moving business area conditions.

Quick prototyping and Least Functional Things (MVPs): Time to feature is principal in novel associations. Spearheading trailblazers ought to embrace least reasonable things (MVP) improvement and quick prototyping. Affiliations can procure client input, immediately test and survey weighty considerations, and further foster their proposals considering certifiable encounters thanks to this iterative method.

Lean Startup technique creates solid areas for interactive development and advancing learning. Venturesome trailblazers should apply lean thoughts, underlining the improvement of a viable game plan through experimentation, affirmed learning, and effective resources for the leaders.

15.2 Adjusting Game plans to Record for Changing Business area Examples
Arranging a strategy around the client:
Strong client care is the principal of a successful business. Game plan setup should take on a client-driven methodology, with an accentuation on the tendencies, torture locales, and approaches to acting of the goal market. This accentuation on the necessities of the purchaser coordinates the development of work and items that are tempted by the goal market.

Flexibility and Flexibility in Strategies: Game plans ought to be versatile and adaptable in erratic business places. Game plans that engage adaptability and progression considering moving business area designs should be made by spearheading pioneers. Researching different income sources, and strategies for dispersing, and banding together frameworks might be central to this.

Open turn of events and headway conditions: Business pioneers should interface with outside advancement organic frameworks. To get to a greater pool of best-in-class considerations and development, this incorporates working with new organizations, universities, gas pedals, and industry specialists. The circuit of resources and capacities from outside the association into its strategy is simplified by open progression drives.

Scaling Undertakings in Shaky Circumstances: Viable Improvement Approaches
Fundamental Intrigues and Associations:

Fundamental plots can offer important resources, entry to new business areas, and further created capacities in volatile settings. Bold supervisors ought to intensely search for open entryways for affiliations and coalitions that improve and reinforce the association's advantages.

Market understanding and data-driven free heading: Spearheading pioneers should use market information and data to coordinate their improvement drives. To do this, you can utilize appraisal, purchaser snippets of data, and horrible assessment to assist you with picking how colossal to scale your business. Advancement drives will undoubtedly be as per client tendencies and market demand when data-driven frameworks are used.

Lean Errands and Resource Headway: In unsteady business places, compelling exercises are critical for the long stretch turn of events. To update utilitarian efficiency, improve resource designation, and smooth out procedures, venturesome trailblazers should take on lean norms. This lean procedure attracts relationships to develop substantially more capably while decreasing waste and extra expenses.

We are doused in the shocking space of undertaking unusual business areas To some degree. Ambitious trailblazers can successfully vanquish weaknesses by embracing swift business, changing strategies to advance examples, and attempting affordable improvement plans. Persistently recollect that the principal ways for venturesome endeavors to win in the constantly moving business scene are through improvement, client focus, and key alliances.

Chapter 16

Investigating Correspondence Hardships

Techniques for Defeating Normal Obstacles

In the powerful scene of expert correspondence, challenges are unavoidable. This part tends to a portion of the normal obstructions people and associations might experience and gives systems to explore them successfully.

16.1 Tending to Mistaken Assumptions and Misinterpretations

Undivided attention and Explanation:

Empowering undivided attention and posing explaining inquiries when there's a potential for error. This ensures that messages are gotten as planned.

Looking for Input:

Effectively looking for input from beneficiaries of correspondence to check their comprehension and recognize regions for development.

16.2 Overseeing Struggle and Conflicts

Keeping up with The ability to appreciate anyone on a profound level:

Utilizing the ability to appreciate anyone on a profound level to move toward clashes with self-restraint and sympathy. This spreads out an exceptional climate for settling contrasts.

Working with Open Exchange:

Making a protected and open space for all gatherings required to communicate their points of view and worries, fully intent on tracking down commonly satisfactory goals.

16.3 Defeating Language and Social Obstructions

Giving Language Backing: Offering language assets and backing for people who might confront difficulties because of phonetic contrasts.

Social Responsiveness Preparing: Giving preparation and assets to improve social mindfulness and awareness, it is conscious and comprehensive to guarantee that correspondence.

16.4 Managing Troublesome Characters

Understanding Conduct Types: Applying conduct-based correspondence procedures to draw in people who might have testing characters.

Defining Limits and Assumptions: Laying out limits and assumptions for correspondence, guaranteeing that cooperation stays useful.

16.5 Overseeing Virtual Correspondence Weakness

Adjusting Coordinated and Non-Concurrent Correspondence: Finding some kind of harmony between ongoing cooperation and nonconcurrent correspondence to forestall burnout and guarantee successful commitment.

Empowering Screen Breaks: Upholding for standard breaks from virtual correspondence stages to decrease weakness and keep up with concentration and efficiency.

16.6 Dealing with Emergency Correspondence

Readiness and Lucidity:

Guaranteeing that emergency correspondence plans are set up, with clear jobs and obligations characterized for all partners.

Straightforwardness and Compassion:

Imparting straightforwardly and compassionately during seasons of emergency, giving convenient updates and consolation to every single included party.

By proactively tending to these normal correspondence difficulties, people and associations can foster versatility and flexibility in their correspondence rehearses. This Thus spreads out an exceptional climate for settling contrasts., and prompts more viable and effective expert communications.

Conclusion

In the great orchestra of human undertaking, successful correspondence arises as the director, directs us toward amicable cooperation and shared accomplishments. Our assessment of direct-based correspondence has enlightened the best way to deal with understanding, connecting, and affecting the different wounds around the craftsmanship of characters that invigorate our lord and individual lives.

Taking apart ways of behaving uncovers a fundamental capacity to get through hindrances, cultivate trust, and draw in the results of a full imagination. We've wandered into regions where social awareness thrives, raising our capacity to win in an interconnected general scene. Through an enduring obligation to learning, criticism, and ceaseless development, we encourage a culture of correspondence greatness that resonates in each trade.

To be sure, even amidst the undeniable hardships, we remain steadfast, persevering in our commitment to overcome hindrances and reinforce our bonds. As we adjust to the

consistently moving flows of correspondence patterns, we jump all over chances to refine our art and intensify our effect.

However, let us not fail to remember that our process doesn't finish up here. It conveys forward as an always developing adventure of refinement and edification. In this powerful milieu, correspondence rises above being a simple device; it is the soul of progress, the impulse for development, and the pith of human association.

With each word verbally expressed, each message passed on, and every relationship sustained, we become draftsmen of our reality, making stories of understanding and molding determination. In dominating conduct-based correspondence, we take on the position not exclusively to explore the intricacies within recent memory yet in addition to lead with reason, compassion, and a steady obligation to common perception.

This is our legacy, cut in the records of human affiliation - a legacy that transcends time, causing an extremely durable engraving on individuals who copy our model. May our processes be set apart by groundbreaking discussions, significant associations, and a heritage that reverberates through the ages, for it is through correspondence that we release the full degree of our capability to reshape the world.